Gerry,
Re Self Hypnoses

Help Yourself to a little More Happiness

Greville Wilday

Copyright © 2020 Greville Wilday
All rights reserved

Cover by bellydraft@blueyonder.co.uk

'Our bodies communicate to us clearly and specifically, if we are willing to listen to them.'

'Every time you don't follow your inner guidance, you feel a loss of energy, loss of power, a sense of spiritual deadness.'

'You create your opportunities by asking for them.'

Shakti Gawain.

'Most times when you follow your inner guidance, you feel a gain of energy, boost of power, and a sense of spiritual awareness.'

Greville Wilday

THE AUTHOR

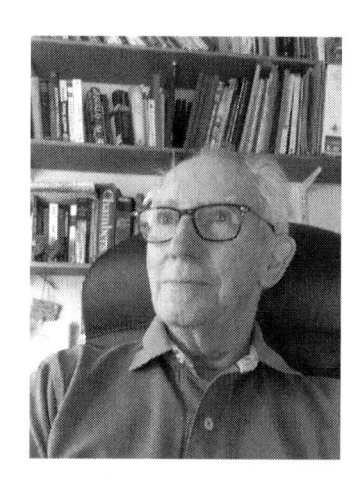

Once he grew out of his dream as a child to be a train driver, Greville Wilday set his heart on becoming a seafarer. Following nautical college and deck apprenticeship, he served as a third officer with a major shipping company. Whilst in port in the West Indies, there was an explosion on his ship. He came to on an operating table under local anaesthetic for surgery on a fractured skull.

Various circumstances, such as the forgoing, have caused him to redirect his life a number of times. A keen student of both people and the world around, he has qualifications in Physics, Computing, Education, Psychological Counselling, and Hypnotherapy. He has lectured to degree level in both Physics and Computing. He has worked as a psychological therapist for many years, including contracts with Greater Manchester Police, ITV, the NHS, and Virgin Trains, as well as helping many private clients.

He has written a number of novels. A county hockey umpire, he is also a keen golfer. He lives on the border of Shropshire and Staffordshire with his wife and a few feline friends.

Books by Greville Wilday

Fiction

Jutland Bank

The Abbey of St. Mary Magdalene

Non-Fiction

Help Yourself to a Little More Happiness

Help Yourself to a Little More Happiness

CONTENTS

Chapter One: Foreword — 1
   Finding your way through this book. — 2

PART ONE: INNER WORKINGS — 3

Chapter Two: Our Internal Guidance System — 4
   Human activity, motivation, and needs. — 4
   A Systems Approach — 6
   Involving Your Conscious Mind — 9
   Switch On! Be Alert! Are you stuck in a loop? — 9
   Be wary of those who tell you what they think you should do! — 10
   Beware of internal voices from others! — 11
   From conscious mind to the subconscious. — 12

PART TWO: MAJOR FACTORS IN WELL-BEING — 14

Chapter Three: Introduction — 15

Chapter Four: Love and Companionship — 18

Chapter Five: Recreation — 21

Chapter Six: Health — 23

Chapter Seven: Exercise — 26

Chapter Eight: Financial Stability and Work/Career. — 27

Chapter Nine: Spirituality and Morality — 29

Chapter Ten: Compassion and Empathy — 31

Chapter Eleven: Flow, Purpose, and Self-Development — 33

PART THREE: ACTIVITIES AND SKILLS TO HELP YOURSELF — 36

Chapter Twelve: Introduction — 37

Chapter Thirteen: Assessing Happiness — 39
   The Nine Major Factors in Well-being — 40

Chapter Fourteen: Managing the Business of Self — 43
   Where to Start — 44
   Planning creatively. — 45
   Getting on with it. — 47
   The Positive Route to Happiness — 47

Chapter Fifteen: Exploring the Way Forward — 49
   The Artist's Date — 50
   Tapping The Subconscious — 50
   Morning Pages — 51
   A Journal — 51
   Basic Word Association — 51
   Drawing on the other side of the brain — 52
   Visual Image Approaches — 52

Chapter Sixteen: Thinking Aids and Examples — 53
   Brainstorming — 53
   Developing the initial ideas further — 54
   Cases Studies for you to try — 57
   Rebecca — 57
   Daniel — 58
   Louise — 59

Chapter Seventeen: Balance: Reduce Distress or Develop Happiness? — 61

Chapter Eighteen: Internal Empowerment and Healing — 63
   Creating a Safe Place — 64
   Anchoring — 65
   Relaxation — 67
   Affirmations — 67
   Self-hypnosis — 68

Chapter Nineteen: Conclusion — 70

PART FOUR: APPENDICES — 71

Chapter Twenty: References and Further Reading — 72

Chapter Twenty-One: Recreative Activities, Hobbies, and Sports — 75

Chapter Twenty-Two: Instructions for self-hypnosis — 80

Chapter One: Foreword

Hi. Thank you for joining me. This is primarily a book to help you to help yourself towards a happier and more fulfilling life. It may also be of value to those whose work is to help others.

So, why is it that you are here? Could it be that life seems fairly good to you, but if it could be improved, would that not be a good idea? Or could it be that you have been struggling with a low mood, feeling unhappy, possibly for some time? Perhaps drugs have been prescribed to help, but things do not seem to be getting much better?

Why should I be able to help you? For several reasons. I have worked as a psychological counsellor, hypnotherapist, and lecturer for many years. This has given me the experience of engaging with many people of a variety of ages and differing backgrounds. It has shown me the power that people have to change their lives and move towards less distress, more happiness, and greater fulfilment. Not surprisingly, at stages in my own life, I have also felt lost, unfulfilled, desperately unhappy, and even suicidal. Finding my way through these experiences, studying therapeutic and personal development, and finding ideas that work, has brought me to sharing these ideas with you.

Our bodies have developed over thousands of years. They have so many wonderful built-in facilities. Sight, hearing, smell, touch, and taste, all help us to keep in touch with the world around us. Memory, feelings, and thoughts help us to process that information. If we cut ourselves within reason, bleeding helps to wash germs out, and healing starts to take place, governed by the body's biological systems. If the dentist removes a tooth it can leave quite a hole, and yet in a relatively few days the gum heals over, and, if we are young enough, another tooth may eventually emerge. So, it should be no surprise that we also have built-in ways in which the mind can help to move us from less healthy unhappiness towards more healthy happiness and fulfilment. Read on and learn how to tap in to these ways.

As with most worthwhile enterprises, the way forward does require some commitment, experimentation, and investment (of time and energy). The rewards can significantly change your life for the better.

Finding your way through this book.

The first chapter, 'Our Internal Guidance System', looks at the way our mind can help us to move forward. It is pretty essential reading. We consider what is going on below the surface.

This is followed by the section introducing the major 'Factors in Well-being', these areas in our lives that have the most effect on generally feeling well or happy.

Next follows a section aimed to help you master 'Activities and Skills to Help Yourself'.

The 'Appendices' contain additional useful information to help you on your way, including further reading.

Advice.

I anticipate that you will enjoy making progress towards where you want to be. Should you feel unduly concerned, it may help to consult a qualified psychological therapist who is a registered member of a professional therapeutic body.

Help Yourself to a Little More Happiness

Part One: Inner Workings

Chapter Two: Our Internal Guidance System

Human activity, motivation, and needs.
Our bodies are continuously active. We have developed with a considerable number of systems that guide our progress, many in a largely automatic way. Consider for example those that fight disease or injury. Medicine and surgical aid can help, but our automatic biochemical responses play a major part. Take another case: suppose that you are at home and want a drink. You walk to where that particular liquid is. To take just a part of that exercise, you do not stop to think about how to move one leg in front of the other. Those procedures are stored in your memory. Of course, it is very different if you are an eight month-old child learning to walk. In many cases our subconscious mind brings stored, learned procedures into play. In some of what we will consider in this book, our conscious mind is brought into play. Sometimes, we need to deliberately engage to try new ways that our mind can learn and then store to replace less helpful old procedures or behaviours.

One of the early researchers into our actions towards well-being, was Abraham Maslow. He approached it from the perspective of human needs, and identified five broad categories:
- Self-actualisation: achieving one's full potential and creativity.

Help Yourself to a Little More Happiness

- Esteem: prestige and feeling of accomplishment.
- Love and belonging: social connections, relationships, intimacy, and friends.
- Safety: personal security, work, resources.
- Physiological: shelter, food and drink, clothing, sex, and rest.

Maslow argued that this was a hierarchy: one aimed to satisfy the more basic needs, such as having food, before being able to do the same with the higher ones such as gaining prestige. Many people these days would see the lower needs as a having priority over the higher ones, without always being required first.

Where the categories seem important to me is that first they highlight that we are all motivated (to engage in human activity), and secondly we can identify areas in which conscious directed activity can improve our sense of well-being.

The following quotation is generally credited to Shakti Gawain, one of the earlier writers on personal development and empowerment, although I cannot find its original source:

'Every time you don't follow your inner guidance, you feel a loss of energy, loss of power, a sense of spiritual deadness.'

I would also argue for a more positive expression:

'Most times when you follow your inner guidance, you feel a gain of energy, boost of power, and a sense of spiritual awareness.'

I use the word 'most', rather than 'every', to recognise that following your inner guidance can sometimes be a testing experience as we come up against new reactions from others, particularly when they have their own agendas.

A systems approach.

What I present next is my estimation of our internal guidance system. I have drawn on my experience in psychological counselling and computer science. The adjacent diagram, 'Conscious Guidance System', represents an automatic system of a type known as a closed loop. Essentially it has: a goal, target, or, in cybernetic language, a 'desired value'; processes causing action or change towards the goal; monitoring of success, and feedback; comparisons; resources to draw on; means of adjusting the action, taken in the light of feedback; and in some cases, a start and finish. In many cases our internal guidance system acts without conscious awareness and choice. However, at times it is desirable for us to weigh up what is going on and make a conscious choice.

Most of the terms in the flowchart boxes are self-explanatory. Several are considered in more depth later in the book. However, it may help to consider a few in a little more detail at this point.

Activity Area refers to an area of human activity, thought, or behaviour. For example, this could be our range of social connections, our thoughts on morality or spirituality, or work.

Within these areas we tend to have goals or aims. In many cases we may not be very aware of these despite their often significant influence. They can be modified consciously and subconsciously. I reckon that many of our initial goals are of genetic origin. As we progress through life we often need to think more deeply about 'what we want', or 'what might be desirable', and modify our goals.

The Activity Repertoire is commonly referred to as the Behaviour Repertoire by psychologists. It is a bit like a wardrobe of possible clothes to put on for various occasions. It includes a number of responses that seem to be genetically hardwired in, like the set of 'fight, flight, or paralysis'. A number of responses, often where intense feelings arise, seem to be drawn on subconsciously, they arise without obvious thought.

Help Yourself to a Little More Happiness

Within the activity repertoire I want to draw your attention to the sources of some learned behaviours. Typically, we tuck away what we have learnt from our parents, teachers, and significant others in our lives, those who you might call 'role models'. We have a strong tendency to behave or react along these learnt routes. Often they are very appropriate, but in some cases they can be destructive and we need to recognise these occasions and choose otherwise. Knife crime, bullying, abusive behaviour, and continuously putting ourselves down are examples. They can be challenged internally by drawing on goals in the morality/spirituality and social connections areas, as well as an awareness of the consequences.

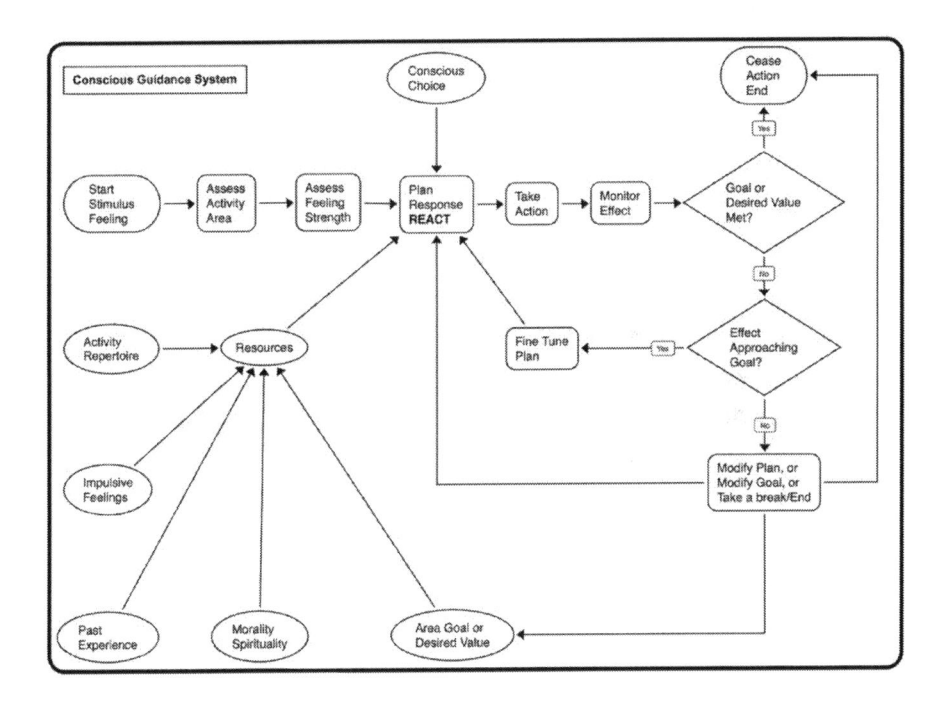

Our Subconscious Internal Guidance System

Let us look a little more deeply at an example of how our hidden subconscious system might work. We can use virtually the same diagram but ignore the Conscious Choice symbol. Suppose you are walking along and there is a loud bang behind you. The stimulus would be the loud sound detected by your ears and possibly other parts of your body. This would be likely to result in an intense feeling of fear. In the REACT process your mind would quickly draw on the area represented by 'Resources' and initially the elliptical symbol to establish the needs Area of Safety. Here a prime Goal is 'staying alive'. From the Activity Repertoire, the prime responses are likely to be 'fight, flight, or paralysis'. Back in the REACT process the plan is likely to be flight, resulting in the Action of moving away quickly. A few seconds later you are likely to appreciate that you are still alive and possibly then stop running away and assess what caused the noise. That sequence is then concluded.

Now consider an example that involves a couple of areas of activity. Suppose that you, your partner or spouse, and young child, live in a flat. A single person lives in the next flat, which is the only other residence in your neighbourhood. It is late evening, and the neighbour knocks on your door.

'I've run out of milk,' the neighbour says. 'Could you lend me some?'

You go to look in your refrigerator and find you have just under half a litre, one pint.

There are a least two Activity Areas involved: the provision of food for yourself and family; and the social connection between you and your neighbour. My estimation is that you would initially draw on the Resources of Past Experience and Morality/Spirituality. If your Past Experience was that the neighbour is an old lady who has difficulty walking but who has often taken in deliveries for you, things would be very different from if it was a selfish young person who frequently made a lot of noise late at night and left a lot of litter around.

The assessment would likely be coloured by the Goal you had in the Social Connection area, it would probably be affected by Compassion and your sense of Morality, and by the Impulsive Feeling you had towards your neighbour.

Help Yourself to a Little More Happiness

To conclude this example, consider the case of the old lady. In searching for what to do, possibly, the Activity Repertoire might suggest offering the old lady a third of a pint in a jug. This helps her and leaves some for your family in the morning. That is the initial Action. It partly meets the Goals you are likely to have for your neighbour and your family. So, possibly, Fine Tuning results in a visit to the supermarket either that evening or next day to purchase milk for your neighbour and yourself.

Involving Your Conscious Mind

Sometimes it is pretty obvious that you need to involve your conscious mind, or weigh up which choice to make. Perhaps, on the way to meet someone, in a town that you do not know very well, you reach a junction with a local council illustrated map displayed. It may be that the map offers two alternative routes of apparently similar length. On closer inspection one route looks to be fairly level and through a shopping area. The alternative can be seen to be devoid of shops but climbs up a steep hill with a fine viewpoint over the surrounding area and a historic castle. Now you have a choice. The outcome would likely be different depending on how keen a shopper you were, whether you were interested in history or architecture, and how fit you were. For some, one factor might dominate. For others, some weighing up might require a more conscious choice.

Switch On! Be Alert! Are you stuck in a loop?

Most of us at some time get stuck in an unsatisfactory loop. This is usually accompanied by a continuing feeling of frustration at the least. For many it shows as a continuing low mood. We want something to improve, or in some cases to go away, and yet we keep doing the same thing, and not surprisingly the adverse feeling, our feedback, continues. In the diagram, we are following the 'No' route from both diamonds but are not taking any action in the following process box. Let me give you two examples.

Consider a young person who has just moved away from home for the first time. They might be a student, have just joined one of the forces, or have moved to take up a new job. Let us say the new venture started a month ago. In any of those positions, the young person might have found it difficult to make friends. The student might be struggling with understanding the lectures and/or doing the course work. In either of the other examples, the young person might be being bullied or find the work very different from what they had expected. The resulting low feeling is an indication from their guidance system that conscious action is needed. The options might include seeking help from the organisation, amending one or more goals, and increasing the level of happiness or satisfaction in an existing happiness area, or starting a new area. The action could involve more than one option.

For a second example, consider someone who has experienced the ending of a relationship by the other person. It would be natural to go through a process similar to grieving and might involve feelings of loneliness, sorrow, anger, and guilt. However, if these feelings seriously persist more than a few weeks, it would be sensible to take some conscious action. Arguably, some action could be taken much earlier.

In all of these cases **our** body is telling us that **we** need to do something. It is a mistake to wait for someone else to come along and fix things for us.

Be wary of those who tell you what they think you should do!

Good parenting and good teaching involves developing in the child or pupil the ability and practice of making sensible choices. In some cases that means exposure to risk and learning to monitor progress in the face of risk. In both parenting and teaching there are times when 'this is what to do' will be appropriate. Outside of these examples for most normal people we need to do what feels right for us. Why?

When another person tells you what they think you should do, they have to be basing this on:

- their perception of the issue, or at the best what they think your perception is,
- their goals, or at the best what they think your goals are,
- their activity repertoire, their library of possible behaviours,
- their past experience,
- their morality/spirituality,
- their feelings,
- and possibly, their ulterior motives.

By all means consider that person's suggestion, but weigh it against what you want to do and what feels right for you. Similarly, if you want to help someone, consider advising or aiding them to explore what they feel is best for them.

Beware of internal voices from others!

In contrast to the fast instinctive response to the loud bang behind, there are occasions when we feel hindered, or restricted in picking our way forward, by internal voices originating in our memory, from other people telling us what to do, and often what not to do. Frequently, these can be in opposition to what we would really like to do. If allowed to dominate without being questioned, these voices can prove destructive and unhealthy.

Consider a student in their first term away from home. Perhaps firm parental and teacher pressure before moving to study away may have continuously emphasised the need to spend a lot of one's own time getting on top of lecture notes and doing lots of examples. I have known many students in this position who found it difficult to take time off to let their hair down and engage in other refreshing activities such as sport, student society, exercise, or meeting with peers to play shove ha'penny in the local pub. Every time they thought of taking a break, an internal voice warned against it. If and when the student did take a break, the relentless voice was present making them feel guilty. Commonly, the student developed a sustained low mood.

As we shall see in the section on factors in well-being, it is wise to be engaged in several areas of human activity and to balance conflicting needs. With students in this position, I usually advised drawing up a weekly timetable that built in time for all essential activities including supporting study/revision, play, and exercise. Then, if the student was playing when they had planned to study, guilt was a useful signal from the guidance system. Additionally, if guilt from internal voices raised itself when in playing time, the timetable was a helpful counter.

As a second example consider a young woman who is living with her mother, where her father has perhaps died young, an only brother has moved away, and the mother is not in good health and is very demanding. It would not be unusual for the young woman in this position to feel frustrated and to develop a sustained low mood. You can perhaps imagine a possible mix of internal and external voices. The young woman's internal guidance system might be pressing for greater fulfilment in areas of self-expression, aspirations at work, play, and companionship. Other voices might be reminding her how mother looked after her when she was a young girl, how poorly mother is, how a good unselfish person ought to be more caring and put mother first, and so on. For the young woman's well-being it is important that she has compassion for herself as well as her mother and that an acceptable solution is found.

From conscious mind to the subconscious.
Your mind is a truly wonderful asset. Consider the toddler struggling to climb to their feet, staggering across a room like an intoxicated person, with apparently little control or grace. Now project that forward to the teenager developing as an artistic ballerina or ballroom dancer, or a gymnast, or a speedy track athlete. By engaging mind and body repeatedly, sophisticated practised procedures have been passed to the subconscious parts of the mind.

Consider the baby who has just a few basic words that parents are so proud of. By the time the child reaches twelve they are likely to have a vocabulary of over ten thousand. A large number of words, with most available quickly, with little conscious thinking. Think about adults who have passed a driving test. At the time of writing, the speed limit on otherwise unrestricted single carriageways is sixty miles per hour. So, drivers in opposite directions are passing each other at a hundred and twenty miles per hour, just a few feet apart, using largely subconscious steering control. My point is that we have exceptionally brilliant internal guidance systems. It can be beneficial to be aware of how to get the best out them.

So much of our behaviour occurs without full conscious awareness. Engage in the business of managing yourself enough and it can become easier. Do it more, then many aspects can become subconsciously automatic. However, it is wise to understand the feedback messages we receive and how to optimise our personal enterprise. These messages commonly occur as feelings, so it is sensible to be tuned in to the emotional side of yourself.

If you are seeking more happiness this will come through developing your engagement and success in areas which are factors in well-being. This may mean areas where you have already made some progress or quite conceivably exploring new areas.

Part Two: Major Factors in Well-being

Chapter Three: Introduction

Now we move on to focus attention on the areas and aspects of life which help to induce a positive mood, a sense of well-being. There has been a lot of research in this area which is surveyed in the excellent book, 'Positive Psychology', by Professor Alan Carr (details in the Appendices). Love and companionship, recreation, health, exercise, financial stability, work, spirituality, compassion, and a sense of purpose are all major factors that can affect our well-being. Our experience and needs in these areas can change substantially as we move through life. Often we can take action to improve a beneficial effect in a given area. In some cases, we can achieve little improvement or even experience a worsening. Then, we can in many cases counter that by taking action in another area. These major factors are developed in this section.

One of the early researchers into increasing happiness arrived at a programme with fourteen fundamentals (Fordyce,1983):

- Be more active and keep busy
- Spend more time socialising and having quality time with other people
- Be productive at meaningful work and pastimes
- Get better organised and plan things out so you accomplish one or two important tasks each day
- Stop worrying because it is unpleasant and unproductive
- Lower your expectations and aspirations, set achievable goals so you will be rewarded by your successes and will be disappointed less often
- Develop positive optimistic thinking
- Get present orientated and live in the moment; don't worry about past hurts or future catastrophes
- Know yourself, accept yourself, like yourself, and help yourself
- Develop an outgoing, social personality and spend time with people you enjoy, and meet new people
- Be yourself and do not disguise who you are, so you will attract people who like you for who you are
- Let go of negative feelings and problems; don't ruminate
- Develop a close romantic relationship
- Value happiness and pursue it with vigour

I mention here, but do not develop further, that vegetation, greenery, countryside, water, and landscape views are often associated with positive feelings. Green decoration is often used in buildings with this in mind. I certainly recall driving home after work in a town and feeling a sense of relaxation spread through me as the view changed from that of a built-up area to that of the countryside. Perhaps you have experienced something similar?

Chapter Four: Love and Companionship

Love is a prime factor in well-being. Through companionship is how it is most often received and expressed. I interpret love and companionship very much more widely than having a few friends. This area of human experience can involve the most intense emotions from self-sacrificial love to murderous hate. For me, it also involves our relationship with ourselves. Yes, there is a significant benefit from being able to accept and get on with oneself. Compassion is an important element within this factor and of sufficient importance for me to treat it separately a little later. Maslow places love and compassion in the centre of his hierarchy of human needs, just above the basic survival factors.

    We can access the benefits of companionship to very varied depths in many different ways. At its most basic, companionship gives us strength and confidence through being accepted. At its best, we are warmed, encouraged, and feel especially valued by loving action from another.

    Close supportive relationships within families and wider social networks are associated with greater well-being, health, longevity, and adjustment. With the exception of those trapped in unhappy marriages, married people tend to be happier than unmarried [see Carr (2011)].

Particularly if we feel lonely, it is worthwhile working to improve our experience of companionship. We can do little to alter the structure of our family, but we can benefit from a wide range of other social networks. We are thrust into networks as school children, students, and at work. Most of us have neighbours and people we meet regularly when we shop. One of the several benefits of religion can be a regular meeting and opportunity for companionship with others. Recreation offers the opportunity to meet with people of similar interests in clubs, sports, hobbies, and a wide range of cultural activities. I will expand on recreation a little later in this section. In addition to humans, a pet can be a warm and wonderful partner in companionship and love. Compassion prompts that we must be ready to care for a pet as a companion. Giving is an important part of companionship.

Whilst companionship is a significant factor in well-being, it is quality rather than quantity that is important. Lots of acquaintances may not be as beneficial as a few good friends. Individuals also vary in their need for company. There seems to be a very wide spectrum here. Some start to feel uncomfortable if they spend long in the absence of company. For others it is just the opposite, they need a fair amount of time on their own. So, if you are generally fairly happy, do not have a large number of friends, and like to have a larger amount of time on your own, there is nothing wrong with this. It is worthwhile spending a little time considering what feels best for you. To a considerable extent this can depend on your personal make-up, and sense of purpose and life goals. These may be factors that you have not given much consideration in the past. They will be addressed in a more detail later.

As mentioned earlier, there is another important aspect of companionship and love, that is living with oneself. Most of us experience periodic negative internal feelings and even voices putting us down, denigrating and trying to convince us that we are worthless or bad in some way.

Most people put a foot wrong on occasion. We then pick up usually uncomfortable feedback responses from either our own morality or spirituality goals, or from others. This is absolutely normal and healthy. It is our internal guidance system trying to help us to get back on track. We then usually have the opportunity to take some corrective action, or may need to adjust our lives as a consequence. If a low mood continues then we need to address that. Expanding action in other well-being areas such as recreation or developing other companionship may well help. If it does not, then it can be wise to seek professional help through a doctor or registered psychological therapist. The chapter on Internal Empowerment and Healing gives other ways of helping oneself in these circumstances.

It may be that you feel you would like more companionship but feel uncomfortable in company and held back. This is quite a common experience. It is a lot easier when you meet with people with a similar interest. This is one of the benefits of having a hobby or activity that regularly brings you into contact with others. The chapter on Recreation develops the theme further. The later chapter on Internal Empowerment may also help with confidence.

Chapter Five: Recreation

Probably one of the most powerful ways to help yourself to a little more happiness is to make sure that you have at least one form of recreation. The word has a Latin derivation. My Cassell's Latin dictionary has 'recreare', the infinitive, as 'to create again, or restore to a sound condition, refresh, invigorate, revive'. These are words which to me beautifully represent the potential of engaging in a suitable recreation.

Call it a hobby, play, or fun, recreation has a sense of freedom and 'letting one's hair down'. Well-being requires us to find some way of giving the little girl or boy inside an opportunity to come out and play. This is even more important if your work is not particularly fulfilling. We all have personal 'wants'. For many, a considerable proportion of our time is spent conforming to society's demands and denying ourselves in some way. Recreation can provide that balancing healthy expression.

Recreation overlaps substantially with other well-being factors. If you engage in a sport as a form of recreation, depending on your choice this may well provide the benefit of exercise. Many sports also necessarily involve regular meeting with others and hence the potential benefit of companionship.

Your recreation might also be an expression of your sense of purpose or spirituality, for example in creating beauty through art, music, or creative writing, or in helping others as a hospital volunteer or Samaritan.

For those who feel that they do not have enough recreation and are wondering what to do, there is a list of activities and hobbies in the Appendices of this book. I suggest that you look through the list and identify a few that might generate a little interest for you. Then give them a few days to incubate before going back to your selection and consider which seems the most appropriate. It may be that you know someone who is involved in your choice. This might provide a route into that particular activity. Many sports or hobbies provide the opportunity to sample them before getting more deeply involved. If, after trying it, your first choice seems disappointing, give it a reasonable go before stopping. Then give it a break before trying something else.

Please see in the Appendices for a table of Recreative Activities and Hobbies

Chapter Six: Health

There seems little doubt that your health can have an impact on how happy you feel. If your health is good it leaves you more free to concentrate on other aspects of life. If your health is poor it can affect your mood and tend to depress. So, it seems pretty obvious that there is a major connection between health and mind. What might not be so obvious is that this works at least three ways. Firstly, poor health can impact on how well you feel and how well your mind works. Secondly, poor health can be picked up by your guidance system to give you messages to improve matters. Thirdly, the mind can be used to improve our perception of health and to improve our health.

In many respects the first and second ways are linked. The adverse feelings of a drop in health are prompts to the internal guidance system to do something. The prime example of this is pain. Pain is usually the body's warning that something is not right and that action needs to be taken. Sometimes this action happens automatically. The sharp feeling experienced in the hand that touches a stinging nettle results in an instinctive movement away by the hand. In other cases, it may be that pain requires professional help by visiting the dentist or doctor. Of course, in some cases there may be no advisable medical remedies and we have to learn to live with pain. This is where some of the other factors in happiness may be able to help. The mind can also assist by the application of relaxation techniques, meditation, or self-hypnosis.

Sooner or later we must all pass away, for some this may be a slow and potentially troublesome process, for others this can happen quickly. However, I am frequently reminded and impressed by the many terminally ill individuals I see or hear about who find some fulfilment in this stage of their lives. They are shining examples of the power of the mind.

For most of us of us, much of the time, we have the opportunity to take action to optimise our health. It pays to take pre-emptive action even though this can be hard work for some. It can save a harder slog over time redressing earlier excesses. It is usually never too late to start to get some benefit. We can help ourselves by taking prudent action in respect of both our body and our mind.

For our body we can help in three main ways: taking care of what goes in, endeavouring to get some exercise (tailored to suit our present state), and acting on internal guidance signals (feelings and related thoughts).

The focus on what enters our body is two-fold: selecting as healthy a diet as we can afford and to some extent tolerate, and avoiding or at least limiting, those things that can damage us. Other texts will advise you better on a healthy diet. I will only comment a little further that alcohol at too high a level in frequency, amount, or strength can do permanent and increasing damage to your liver, heart, and brain. The sooner you act to limit the damage, the better. Drugs, other than those prescribed, can likewise do lasting damage to body and brain. As with alcohol it can be hard work, but not impossible, to come off these.

We can help ourselves to a healthier body and a happier mind by exercise. If you want the detail of proof see Carr (2011). Exercise can release endorphins which tend to make us feel well. Almost whatever your state of health some form of exercise can be tailored to you. Don't wait for someone else to tell you. Start to explore for yourself!

As always, we can tune in to our internal guidance system. This may be through its prompts such as 'That sport, or activity, looks fun'. Take it a little further and find out how you might get involved.

Chapter Seven: Exercise

As we discussed in the chapter on health, some form of exercise, or indeed more than one, can contribute to our sense of well-being. It helps to keep the body healthy, can release the endorphins which make us feel good, give pride in personal achievement, and bring us companionship.

For those with a reasonable degree of fitness, exercise might be through a sport. Don't worry if exercise makes you think of P.E. at school, and perhaps you didn't enjoy it. If you enjoy gym workouts, that's great. I never have. But I have enjoyed a number of sports. Dancing, with its many forms, appeals to a lot of people. For those who are virtually chair bound, there are sets of exercises that one can do. Indeed, some can be to music which can make them even more fun. Start to experiment.

Depending on your current fitness and health you can choose where to enter the wide scale of activities and sports. Starting at exercises of the limbs when sitting down, one can move through, walking, dancing, playing bowls, golf, jogging, up to the more energetic activities such as athletics, badminton, football, hockey, rugby, or tennis. For more ideas, please look at the list of activities and hobbies in the Appendices.

Chapter Eight: Financial Stability and Work/Career.

Many people assume that if they were wealthier, then they would be happier. Research shows that this is by no means always true. Carr (2011, p23), summarises a considerable amount of study in this area and concludes that: 'Unless they are very rich, people who strive for wealth are less happy than those who aspire to non-material goals and values'.

What seems more fundamental to me is being financially stable, where income at least slightly exceeds expenditure, and at least basic needs are met. In my estimation, many people would be happier if they spent less money on inessentials, and focussed more attention and energy on one or more non-material goals and activities that appealed to them. Ideally, some of these would be in-line with their core aims and values.

So, if you are of working age and reasonably fit, having a job that brings in enough income is an important factor in happiness. That brings us on to the topic of the work itself. You are likely to be happier in work or a career that you identify with and that matches your skills, intelligence, and aptitudes. Ideally, work can be a fulfilment of one or more of our aims. Then it can also become a means of self-expression and rewarding in the non-monetary sense.

In the area of work, most people will at some time get adverse feedback messages or feelings ranging through disappointment, fear, loneliness, a sense of being unfairly treated, to anger and hate. I found an interesting article on this topic on the BBC News website, Ascher (2019). Often this problem can be resolved by discussion with an appropriate person, perhaps the manager in question, if that feels comfortable. In cases of bullying or harassment, this is probably best raised with HR. The topic of satisfaction and happiness at work should be a major one for any enterprise, if only from the perspective of maximising productivity. Employees who are unhappy are likely to be less effective. If the issue is unresolved, the employee may choose to take their talents and skills elsewhere, with the consequent cost of advertising and training for their replacement.

For those who have a job that brings in for them an acceptable income, and where desired advancement appears to be out of reach, self-expression, and sometimes increased income, may be found within one or more other activities. I can recall many people who have developed part-time activities such as local politics, amateur dramatics, running a dance school, and offering hairdressing, after appropriate training.

Of course, not everyone is of an age or fitness to work. That is one less factor in improving happiness. All the more reason to consider the others.

What emerges from this, is that it is very worthwhile to periodically spend a little time assessing your aims and values, auditing your degree of happiness and fulfilment, and weighing up what action you might take towards greater happiness.

Chapter Nine: Spirituality and Morality

Spirituality is about making sense of our place in the physical and social universes. One of the ways that people do this is through religion, belief in a God. For others, it is accepting that there is no God and that life is finite. Either way, it is about coming to terms with existence and resolving natural fears around this. A basic goal is 'staying alive'. We need to come to terms with sooner or later being unsuccessful!

Those with regular religious practices tend to be happier than those who don't (Myers et al., 2008). This can be for several reasons including companionship.

Associated with spirituality and religion is morality. This is concerned with distinguishing between good and bad behaviour, right and wrong. This has an effect on happiness in that it affects how we are perceived by others, and that can affect how we feel. Most people wish to be liked and respected by others and find that this tends to improve their self-esteem and well-being. Being moral brings benefits. Characteristics that are regarded as positive include honesty, compassion, fairness, and generosity. Negative characteristics include greed, laziness, unkindness, selfishness, and aggressiveness. See Hartley, A. (2016).

This is a factor that can affect well-being in polar opposite directions. A strongly-held moralistic approach associated with an overtly judgemental regard of others, a lack of compassion and empathy, and a readiness to force one's views on others, has led to much cruelty and unhappiness in the past and present. I put this down to the absence of love and compassion. Whereas, a morality or spirituality based on love can produce profound outward-directed goodwill, well-being in self and others, and a better acceptance of oneself.

So, you might well ask, how does one approach thinking about those who behaviour is contrary to our system of morality? This is a common challenge to therapists. The answer, which is well tried and tested but often hard work, is to practise separating the behaviour from the person. You learn to disagree or dislike the behaviour, whilst trying to empathise with and understand the individual. When you look into it more deeply, you often find that an abuser has themselves been a victim of abuse.

Compassion and empathy seem to me to be fundamental bedrocks of morality and happiness. We consider these further in the next chapter.

Chapter Ten: Compassion and Empathy

Compassion and empathy are attributes that tend to help in the formation and maintenance of relationships (de Waal, 2008). Relationships, including with oneself, are a major factor in happiness. Thus, it is worthwhile endeavouring to develop these attributes, if you wish to increase your happiness.

Compassion is a feeling of care for another person and tends to imply a need or suffering by the other person. Compassionate people tend to have developed the attributes of altruism, forgiveness, gratitude, and humility. Altruistic motivation is defined by the intention of improving another person's situation, for that reason alone, and not for ulterior self-serving motives (Carr, A. 2011. p282). Such a person would perform a caring deed without needing to have others become aware of it. To me, it is an example of unselfish love. Perhaps strangely, although not intended, it can provide an emotional reward to the giver.

Empathy is the ability or act of endeavouring to be aware of the feelings of another person. To help develop empathy it can be beneficial to reflect on the effect that our behaviour might have on others.

Working to develop the previously instanced attributes of compassion and empathy can be therapeutic. It can help to reduce distress and improve a sense of well-being.

Focussing some of your attention on the good things in your life, can help to develop gratitude and a sense of ease and joy. Whereas, if you spend time focussing on the less satisfactory things in your life, you are likely to experience low mood. Take all the opportunities that come your way to express and develop gratitude. That extra step, a word or note of thanks, will help not only yourself but also the person you express it to. Take time each day to be aware of the good things that you have experienced. Say 'thanks' to your God or to your good fortune.

When you have suffered in some way due to the actions of another person, festering or suppressed anger can eat away at happiness. At times, you might improve matters by discussion with the other person, particularly if the other person endeavours to ameliorate the matter. Letting it go, with forgiveness, can help you relax internally. This takes a lot of practice and is well worth the effort.

The converse can also help reduce distress or improve happiness. Can you accept that you are wrong? You may find that accepting that you have caused hurt to someone else, whilst perhaps assessing this as unintended, can help move a disagreement forwards. A genuine apology or restitution, is an example of a compassionate considerate person. It usually increases respect.

Both forgiveness and contrition can be very hard work. They involve humility. However, they can help to develop goodwill and happiness.

It may seem strange, but developing compassion towards, and empathy with, others, can help to develop a happier person in oneself.

Chapter Eleven: Flow, Purpose, and Self-Development

In this chapter, I delve deeper into what seem to me to be the fundamentals of a more fulfilling, satisfying, and usually happier life.

When people are most fulfilled, at least periodically, and sometimes frequently, they are deeply engaged in an activity. This experience was named 'flow' by the psychologist who has probably studied it most, Professor Mihaly Csikszentmihalyi.

When a person is experiencing flow, they are intensely absorbed in what they are doing, and are temporarily unaware of other aspects of self and their surroundings (Carr, A. 2011, p133). Usually they experience satisfaction, enjoyment, or happiness, sometimes intensely.

The requirement for flow is an activity in which the person:

- is engaged in a task, and
- the task presents a challenge, and
- the challenge is matched to the person's skill level, and
- there is feedback, and

- the person experiences a sense of control, and
- the person is intrinsically motivated, that is they do the activity because they like it.

Examples of flow occur in computer games, creative writing, hobbies, making or listening to music, painting, sex, socialising, sport, study, watching films, and work, (Csikszentmihalyi, 1997).

Shernoff and Csikszentmihalyi (2009) concluded that the following approaches in education facilitate flow experiences and lead to better academic and behavioural outcomes:

- making learning enjoyable, and
- making learning challenging in a way that matches task challenges with pupils' level of skill.
- Once again this requires tapping in to intrinsic motivation.

Flow at work occurs when workers have a sense of control over their jobs, where their jobs require use of well-developed skills to do challenging tasks, and they have clear goals and receive frequent feedback (Csikszentmihalyi, 2003).

A further general point was revealed by Csikszentmihalyi. As skill level rises it is found that the challenge level needs to rise for flow to happen. Also, as most people experience, if our skill level is not quite high enough and we frequently do not succeed in the challenge, then we need to pick a slightly lower challenge. Otherwise we can feel dispirited: our guidance system is providing feedback suggesting a need for change.

Overall, we need to be a little careful. It seems on the surface that flow might be a universal ambrosia. However, flow in computer games can lead to an addiction. So can sex and work. Crime, burglary and rape can all give an intense engagement and flow. Unhappiness can then result through depression, imprisonment, and becoming a social outcast. Balance and common sense in life's endeavours, and relation to a spiritual and moral background appear to be important.

Taking these ideas forward, at its simplest it is worthwhile having a hobby activity that you enjoy. We can also learn from the fact that flow is related to having a goal in that area or activity. From this it seems that it is very helpful to have a personal periodic assessment of the factors that contribute to a sense of well-being. Do you need to make any changes?

Further, and probably most fundamental to me, we need to periodically ask ourselves what we want from life. What are your most fundamental desires? Unless you are working towards these in some way, you are likely to experience at least some periods of dis-satisfaction. If you can build into your life some activity or movement for self-expression of your highest aims, or Purpose, you can experience what Maslow called self-actuation and feel in tune with yourself.

As we move on through life we need to periodically stop and take stock. Sometimes our desires prove to be unattainable, or new opportunities open up. Then we need to plan afresh.

If you are able to find work that is closely related to your most significant aims or motivation in life, then your work has the potential to be satisfying, fulfilling, and self-expressive.

For some, identifying what you want from life is not straight forward and might take time to develop. When you have discovered what you want from life, then the motivation starts and you need to set some goals to give prudent direction and help progress. The chapters in the next section are designed to help here.

Part Three: Activities and Skills to Help Yourself

Help Yourself to a Little More Happiness

Chapter Twelve: Introduction

Now you know a lot about what affects your sense of happiness and well-being. What do you do with it? This section aims to help you to apply the ideas to help yourself or others.

Firstly, how might you stock-take or assess **your** happiness or well-being? Not surprisingly, this is covered in the next chapter, 'Assessing Happiness'.

'Managing the Business of Self' presents ways of taking this forward and developing a plan of action.

For many people there will remain a sense of '*I have not quite got this right*', until they tune in to the heart of the matter, their sense of Purpose. For some, this can take a while to emerge or be revealed. For many, this will change with time. Techniques, for revealing your deepest aspirations are discussed in the chapter 'Exploring the Way Forward'.

The chapter on 'Examples and Thinking Aids' considers some creative and analytical aids and gives a worked example of moving forwards. Three other case studies are provided for readers to apply their ideas.

For most of us, at some time distress will hit hard. The question of whether to endeavour to increase happiness at this time is addressed in the chapter 'Balance: Reduce Distress or Increase Happiness'.

The final chapter, 'Internal Empowerment and Healing' provides a number of techniques to help yourself on your journey towards greater happiness and fulfilment.

Chapter Thirteen: Assessing Happiness

How happy are you? Most of us don't stop to think about this until our guidance system forces us to recognise that we have a sustained low mood. For many, the next step is a course of antidepressants. What a shame! The body is giving us a prompt to do something, and we take action to suppress the prompt. A referral for counselling would frequently be more appropriate. Better still would be to use our own brain to assess the issue and negotiate our way forward towards what our whole person wants.

    What I would suggest is a regular appraisal of how happy we are. Failing this, do it when your mood tells you that things could be better. Explore how you feel about the nine factors that have been discussed in the previous section and are listed below. You may find that you have never really thought about some. Of course, for some people they will be able to do little about one or more factors. If your health is poor and you are well past retirement age you may be able to little about exercise or work. However, although confined to a chair, some arm or upper-body exercise may be possible and can be made even more beneficial when done to music.

For many people, two or more factors may be related. Limited opportunity to progress at work can fire energy towards other areas. For some, this might be expressed in exercise or recreation such as sport, dancing, or amateur dramatics. For those with more developed levels of spirituality or compassion it might lead to voluntary work. For those with a strong altruistic feeling this might develop their sense of purpose to move towards a caring profession or voluntary work.

The Nine Major Factors in Well-being
- Love and Companionship
- Recreation
- Health
- Exercise
- Work/Career
- Financial Stability
- Spirituality and Morality
- Compassion and Empathy
- Purpose in Life

Happiness Assessment Method
The approach is essentially subjective:

1. Consider, in turn, each of the nine major factors in well-being and rate how satisfied and clear you are in each, out of 10. Thus: 0 means you are totally dissatisfied, 10 means you are totally satisfied and things could not be better.
2. Draw these estimations on a rough block graph as in the example below.
3. Consider which factors you could do something about. Some may feel more important or urgent than others.
4. The following chapters give help in taking matters forward.

5. Periodically review.

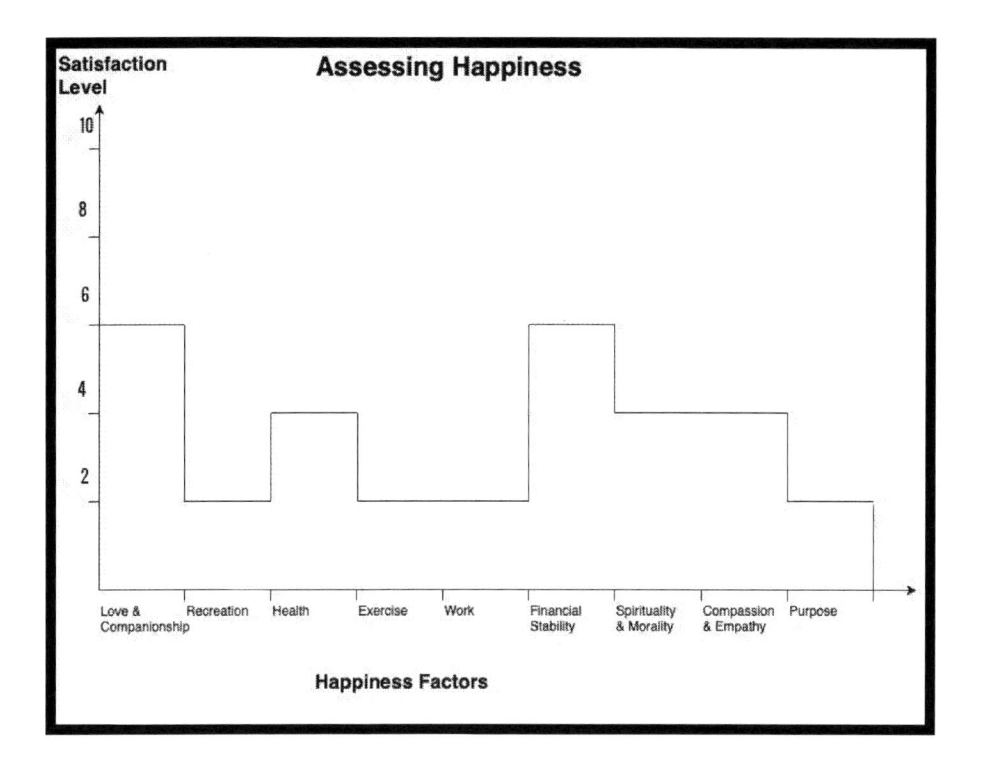

Assessing Happiness

Happiness Factor	Satisfaction Level
Love & Companionship	5
Recreation	1
Health	3
Exercise	1
Work	3
Financial Stability	5
Spirituality & Morality	3
Compassion & Empathy	3
Purpose	1

The above chart is for a thirty-year-old single male. He lives alone and has parents, siblings, a few friends, and a girl-friend. He does little in the way of recreation except watch TV. His health is not great: he is overweight and has diabetes related to this. He does not fancy exercise other than to take his parents' dog for an occasional walk. He does not find his work engaging or enjoyable, but it brings in what he feels is a satisfactory income. He has never thought much about life in general, what he wants from it, or to give to it. He sees himself as fairly tolerant and good-natured. He would admit that he is just drifting along at present.

You might like to think about what he could try if he wanted to make his life happier?

Here are some of my thoughts. Firstly, any action needs to be his choice, based on what seems important to him. For a number of people, the Spirituality factor drives Purpose. This might work through as a desire to help, or create. Where there is a strong desire like these, it is ignored at peril. For some people, a sense of purpose arises only with time. Our young man might do well to reflect on what sort of work he would LIKE to do. Then, he needs to weigh up what training would be required and how he feels about that. He might decide it was too hard to go down that route and instead look for some self-expression in a sport or recreational hobby. If he could find a sport or exercise that he enjoyed, that would help his health.

Further examples may be found in the chapter 'Thinking Aids and Examples'.

Now! What about yourself?

Chapter Fourteen: Managing the Business of Self

In many respects, a person is rather like a business enterprise. We have desires, opportunities, competition, problems, threats, costs, and so on. I was involved in helping a number of small businesses at one time and was surprised at the considerable variety of thought that the owners would put into running their businesses. It varied from a lot, to minimal. I was surprised to find that some would not bring their accounts to a reasonable overview until after the end of their trading year. Thus, a problem or an opportunity could have been developing unknown for several months. Not surprisingly a number of organisations go out of business every year.

Perhaps you don't really see yourself as comparable with a business. Just consider a few figures, purely from the point of view of finance, which is certainly not the most important human consideration. At the time of writing, the UK Office for National Statistics gives the median employed person's annual salary as about £30,000. Over the course of say fifty years' work, that person would earn £1,500,000, assuming they stayed at the same real value of income as at the time of writing. That is a significant total for many people. As I have pointed out earlier in this book, financial stability is only one of several factors in well-being, or happiness.

So, how YOU run YOUR Business of Self is worth some consideration. You are the business chairperson, managing director, accountant, production director, purchasing director, human resources director, creativity person, and, of course, tea boy or girl. Why not take a few leaves out of the books of successful companies.

You possess an excellent guidance system that will help. It will give you feedback, largely via mood, on how your business is going. But you need to supply periodic, or even regular, occasions to assess and direct progress (board meetings). You also need times to reflect on where the business is going and where you would like it to go. Many organisations give this the grand title of Mission Statement. It is comparable with what I have called Purpose. What do you want from life? What do you want to give to life? How do you go about achieving satisfaction, application, enjoyment, fulfilment, happiness, flow?

Where to Start

It is worthwhile spending a little time taking stock and assessing whether you have any burning ambitions waiting to be fulfilled. A significant help is to be alert to your Wants as opposed to your Shoulds. Work through your well-being factors considering especially those where you assess a lower level of satisfaction. Also consider whether you are getting enough self-expression. Are you providing sufficient opportunity for the little girl or boy within to come out and play? Is there enough fun and pleasure in your life? Are you getting the creative or artistic expression that feels right? Do you need more education towards better fulfilment in your career or a hobby?

This is initially a time for divergent thinking. Identify a few areas, say three or four, with potential for, and interest or desire in development. Avoid going into each in depth at this stage. This is a time for brain-storming.

Following is a list of areas to think about, the order of importance will differ from person to person. One or more may stand out to you.

Areas to consider

- Love and Companionship
- Recreation
- Health
- Exercise
- Work-Career
- Financial Stability
- Spirituality and Morality
- Compassion and Empathy
- Purpose in Life
- Artistic or other creative expression
- Education
- Recreation
- Pleasure

Planning creatively.
From your three or four areas select one and decide on a goal. Write this down in clear words. This is where you want to end up after planned activity. It needs to be something clearly achievable and measurable. Some examples might be:

- To pass grade four in piano,

- To be promoted to the position of supervisor,
- To pass my car driving test,
- To ask someone out for a date,
- To get selected for the third team,
- To start my own business,
- To join The Samaritans.

In deciding which one of the, say, four areas to work on, it can be helpful to draw up a list of pros and cons for each.

Break down your goal into sub-goal steps.
You may need to acquire resources or knowledge. Some steps need to be taken before others. Passing grade four in piano would need the use of a piano, probably piano lessons, one or more music books, possibly you might choose to pass a lower grade first. Each of these is a step or sub-goal on the way to achieving your goal. Some may need to be done before others, some can overlap or be done at the same time.

If you are planning to start your own business you may need to:

- run it in parallel with your current job for a while,
- enrol on a course of basic accounting
- develop a business plan,
- research/acquire premises,
- acquire more tools or equipment,
- get some advice on marketing and advertising,
- Plan an appropriate sequence of tasks.

Help Yourself to a Little More Happiness

Getting on with it.
Once you have committed yourself to your goal and done any necessary planning it is prudent to keep an eye on how things are going. Monitor your progress and learn from the 'feedback'. Few people achieve their goals without some hiccups. Don't be put off by the first setback. On the other hand, it may well be that things go surprisingly well and your enthusiasm is soon rewarded.

Achieving one's goals is a bit like a journey. From our starting point, which has a good view, we plan our route towards a distant town. For part of the way the traffic is light and the surrounding countryside is beautiful. Then we find our intended route is blocked or severely restricted. That is not necessarily a major problem. We modify our plan and take a slightly different route. If it turns out that the town we wanted to pass through has its market day on the day we chose, we tuck that information away for our benefit in the future.

So, with the benefit of feedback from monitoring, we sometimes need to modify our plan.

The Positive Route to Happiness
For many of our goals, there will be the joy en route of being and feeling in tune with ourselves. Making a conscious effort to be positive, confident, and cheerful can both help us feel good and rub off on those we meet along the way.

Some set-backs are inevitable. It is beneficial to learn from these and to not let ourselves become dispirited. You, I, have the choice as to whether we let low mood depress us. It is purely a feedback to make some change. Consider a young baby learning to walk! Most will stagger a few steps and then totter and collapse. They don't give up. They try again, often experimenting with alternatives. They frequently scramble on all fours to begin with. Then, with a hand on adjacent furniture, they manage many more steps. Some-time later they may turn out to be elegant and graceful dancers, fleet of foot athletes, or just ordinary happy people getting on with life's ups and downs.

Inevitably, in some cases it is clear that we will not, or do not, achieve our intended goal. This can seem a setback. It is prudent to regard the inevitable feelings as a feedback from our guidance system to make a change. Changing the route may not be possible. This is when we need to be aware that there are many other places worth travelling to on our way to happiness and fulfilment. Review your happiness factors and consider other goals. As I have mentioned before, I know of many people who found themselves limited in their desired career progress. Most found fulfilment though other routes. Some devoted more time to public service, others to hobbies or sport, and yet others to starting their own businesses. Our minds are full of wonderful healing and self-expressive resources. Tune in and let yours help you.

Chapter Fifteen: Exploring the Way Forward

For a number of people, despite making progress towards happiness, there remains a nagging uncertainty. Commonly, this is about concern over their major direction in life, or Purpose. What do you want from life? What do you want to give to life?

Frequently, this has a spiritual or moral involvement. Sometimes, the central or dominant drive takes a while to clearly emerge, but can be helped by a number of techniques that encourage the subconscious to speak through. Sometimes, we need to recognise that the 'shoulds' of morality, that appear to be dominating, are those of past significant others telling us what they think we should do. Whilst those might have a place in the background, it is important to also be aware of our own needs and wants. It is important for our psychological well-being that our own aspirations and desires are recognised and honoured in some way.

In moving forward, I address the last idea first. For many people, the thought of spending time or energy on themselves appears selfish. Let me assure you that it need not be. If you are well and happy in yourself, you will be in a much better position to help others. As the politicians love to say, 'Let's be clear', I am not suggesting that you devote all your energy to yourself. No! Compassion and empathy have important roles to play in developing happiness. However, as I have suggested before, it is important also to nurture yourself. Let the little girl or boy within come out to play and develop their own creativity and happiness.

The Artist's Date

A good way to start is to regularly plan an 'Artist's Date' for yourself on a weekly basis. The idea is discussed at greater length in the excellent book, 'The Artist's Way', by Julia Cameron (Cameron 2016). This book is not specifically for visual artists, but treats all individuals as being artists and creative in some form, and helps to develop expression and self-confidence. The artist's date is a block of time set aside regularly to spend on nurturing yourself. It is specifically for you on your own. It might be a couple of hours spent on a walk, playing the piano, or just relaxing in a cafe. It is for you to choose. You will be learning to be more at ease with yourself and open to emerging ideas.

Plan Your Artist's Date on a regular basis.

Tapping The Subconscious

I mentioned our subconscious when considering our internal guidance system, pointing out how it can store away many different forms of behaviour ready to be called into action at a prompt. In addition to this, the mind seems to work away behind the scenes to make sense of various aspects of life. One of those aspects is our deepest motivation and need for expression, or purpose. Since most of our thinking is done via words, the access to our deepest thoughts and ideas is also via words for most people. This is commonly through the way our minds associate or link words and ideas. Some ways of accessing your subconscious are now revealed.

Help Yourself to a Little More Happiness

Morning Pages
This is a second idea from Cameron(2016). You need a blank book and a pen or pencil, that is all. Then, every day you set aside some time to write three pages of what-ever comes into your head. This is called 'stream of consciousness' writing. Parts of it will seem strange and almost nonsense. The pages are not intended to be clever. They will often appear to be negative or kitchen sink in content. They are a form of meditation. Sooner or later, ideas that are important to the person who writes, start to emerge.

A Journal
For a number of people, a more standard journal can provide a way for innermost thoughts to emerge. This will initially tend to be a record of what has happened on each day. If you let this expand to include thoughts, feelings, assessments, and wishes, then patterns and motivations can start to appear.

Basic Word Association
A shorter approach to inner motivations is basic word association. For this, you need a blank sheet of say A4 paper and a pen or pencil. Do it somewhere quiet and on your own. At the top left of the paper write, with your normal writing hand, the first word or brief phrase that comes into your head. Focus on this word or phrase, and write the next word that comes into your head. Repeat this procedure for two minutes, separating each next word by a comma (,) and writing normally in lines. Then fold up the paper, on a row by row basis, so as to hide each preceding day's writing.

Each following day, do this again, starting on the next blank line, without looking back at the previous day's writing. Do this for a week, then put the paper, or papers, away for a week.

Finally, unroll the paper and read what you have written. It is surprising how often significant words or phrases arise when you look back. These can often suggest important motivations or interest to you.

Drawing on the other side of the brain

Now try the immediately prior basic word association exercise but use the opposite hand to your normal one for writing. This accesses the other side of the brain, the opposite to the one you are writing with. In this way you will have accessed both sides of your brain drawing on quite different natural functions. You may find this slow and hard work at first, but it usually improves as you do it more.

Visual Image Approaches

For those who are more visually artistic, a notebook of doodles and sketches can help to develop creativity and reveal aspirations. There are several books which can help you with ideas, routes, exercises, and interpretations: Capacchione(2002), Edwards(1993), and Edwards(1988).

Chapter Sixteen: Thinking Aids and Examples

This chapter gives a few examples of exploring the way forward, starting with the young man we considered in the earlier chapter on Assessing Happiness. This is a worked example which represents my thinking. Three cases are provided for you to try your hand, bringing your approach to life.

It helps to write things down in some form, both as a record and because seeing an idea can often lead subconsciously to another related one. For people who do a lot of thinking, either creatively or analytically, there are a number of computer programmes or 'apps' that can help. Lists and diagrams can both be used. If you like lists, then bulleted points in a word processing program can offer the opportunity to tidily amend or add in a hierarchical way.

Brainstorming

Starting with brainstorming, our young man might look through the list of areas to consider, assess the low points in his graph as starting places, and come up with something like the following. In brainstorming, the approach is to come up with as many different ideas as possible without digressing to develop any of them. He might jot them down as a list:

Improving my happiness
- Work ?
- Exercise
- Hobby
- Self-Expression.

Or he might prefer to represent his ideas graphically, as in the following diagram.

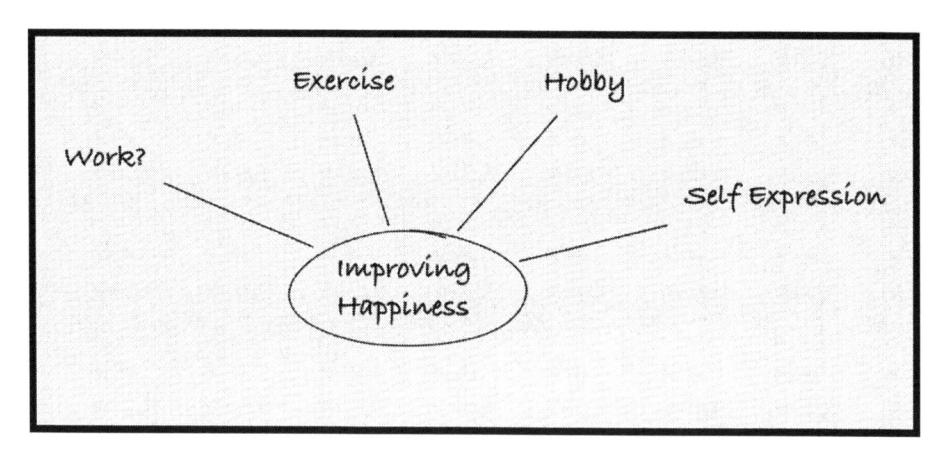

Brainstorming Diagram Example

Developing the initial ideas further
Before deciding which route to go down, quite probably our young man might want to develop his thoughts along each of the

branches he has identified. Using the bulleted list approach, he might end up with something like the following:

Improving my happiness
- Work ?
  - Now, car assembly line
  - Making things
  - Liked carpentry at school
- Exercise
  - With others
  - Cycling
    - Join club
      - Get fitter first
      - Riding on my own
    - Clothing
- Hobby
  - Making models
    - Wood based
      - Course?
- Self-Expression
  - On stage?
    - Am Dram
      - Scenery start
  - Music
    - Guitar
      - Lessons
    - Choir
  - Create
    - Design
      - Course

Using the graphical approach, it might come out like this:

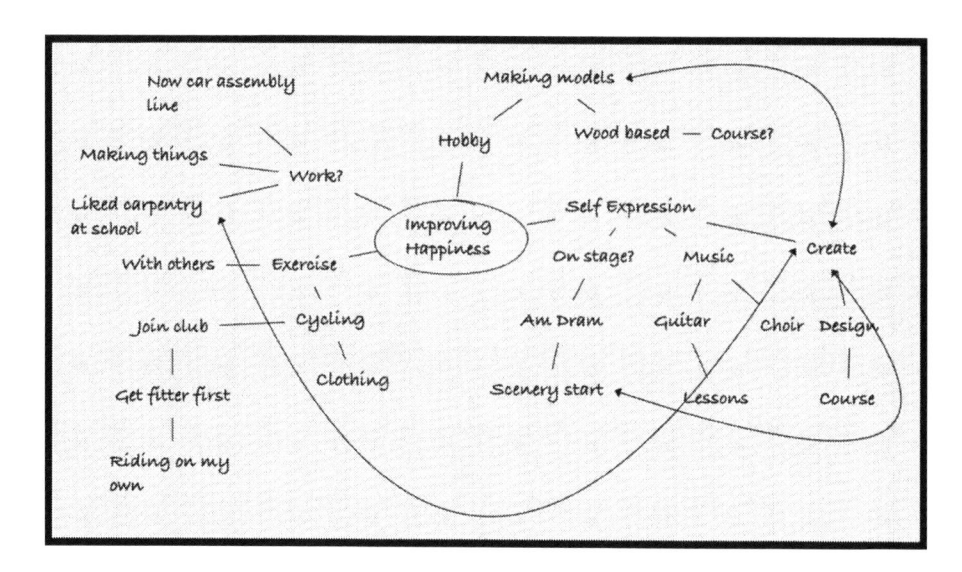

```
Now car assembly                Making models
line                              /        \
   \                           Hobby     Wood based — Course?
Making things  \                /
           \   Work?     
Liked carpentry  \      Improving     Self Expression
at school          \    Happiness    /      \
  With others — Exercise   /      On stage?   Music      Create
              \       /         /         \      \    /
  Join club — Cycling      Am Dram       Guitar  Choir  Design
      |         \            /              \       |
  Get fitter first  Clothing  Scenery start — Lessons   Course
      |
  Riding on my
  own
```

Idea Development Mind Map

The development from the original brainstorm has been displayed above in a form called a Mind Map. This was popularised by psychologist Tony Buzan in a BBC TV program. He wrote an excellent book: 'Use Your Head'. My current edition was published in 2006 (see References).

The bulleted list approach that I used earlier is, technically, a hierarchical or tree structure. If you remove the curved relationship lines from the mind map this would give the same structure in a graphical format. The originating node, Improving Happiness, is known as the root. You can see the first branches emerging, these were the original brainstorm. In turn, these give rise to more branches. One of the many advantages of mind maps is that you can draw on links between branches resulting in a structure known as a network.

Mind maps are very useful aids for developing ideas, for analysis, and for note taking. As well as drawing on paper or other flat surface, there are a number of computer programs or apps. I have listed two in References. The program that I have used is called iThoughtsX.

How might this progress for our young man? It's somewhat like the old question: 'How do you eat an elephant?' Answer: 'A bit at a time'. Don't bite off too much. Don't try to do too many things at the same time. From my perspective, I could see him looking for a model-making design and technology course, part-time. He might learn to make models in different materials. There might even be opportunities for learning and employment within his existing company. You might see things from a completely different perspective, There is no one correct answer. However, it is important to start moving towards what he wants.

Cases Studies for you to try

Try to put yourself in the position of these people and explore what you might consider to increase your happiness. There is no 'Right' answer. Each of us brings a whole different background to what might be appropriate.

Rebecca

Love and Companionship. Rebecca is a nineteen year-old student. She is a member of a happy family and had lots of friends at school. In term time she lives away from home in hall as a university student doing Business Studies. In her second term, she feels quite lonely. She rates this area as 2.

Recreation. She does not get much time for recreation as she spends a lot of time studying to keep up with lectures and course work. She rates this area as 0.

Health. She regards herself as physically fit, but anxious and lonely. She rates this area as 4.

Exercise. She used to play hockey at school, but the only exercise she gets now is walking to lectures. She rates this area as 1.

Work/Career. She thinks she does not have time for a part-time job. She is not too sure of what to do after university and thought a Business Studies course was the safest option. She rates this area as 1.

Financial Stability. Money is tight on a student loan and her family are not well off. She rates this area as 1.

Spirituality and Morality. She thinks that she is a moral person. She rates this area as 2.

Compassion and Empathy. She feels she cares about people. She rates this area as 4.

Purpose. She is not all clear about what she wants from, or to put into, her future. She expects that she will try to get a 'business' job, but is uncertain as to what type. She rates this area as 0.

Daniel

Love and Companionship. Daniel is forty-five, married, with two children, aged sixteen and eighteen. His wife returned to nursing two years ago. He rates this area as 5.

Recreation. His only recreation now is watching television. He rates this area as 1.

Health. He rates his physical health as OK, although he has an enlarged prostate. However, he is depressed over his unemployment and financial situation. He rates this area as 2.

Exercise. He used to play cricket and football regularly until he started a family. He also had a gym membership but has cancelled it to reduce his outgoings. He rates this area as 3.

Work/Career. He was a department store middle manager who was made redundant when his store closed two months ago. So far, he has been unsuccessful in finding another job. He rates this area as 1.

Financial Stability. He is worried about their mortgage and having his elder child due to start university shortly. He rates this area as 1.

Spirituality and Morality. He considers himself to be moral and rates this area as 3.

Compassion and Empathy. He sees himself as a caring person, although he is aware that he has been rather irritable recently. He rates this area as 2 at present.

Purpose. He sees himself as a caring, people person and would really prefer a job that is benefitting others. He rates this area as 3.

Louise
Love and Companionship. Louise is seventy. Her husband died two years ago. Her two children married and moved away from her area. The nearest is fifty miles away. She has four grand-children between them. The children keep in touch. Louise speaks to, and is friendly with, several neighbours. She rates this area as 4.

Recreation. She listens to the radio quite a lot and watches TV. She rates this area as 4.

Health. One hip troubles her at times and she has some arthritis. She rates this area as 4.

Exercise. Shopping is really the only exercise that she gets. She rates this area as 2.

Work/Career. She is a retired secretary. She rates this area as 0.

Financial Stability. She has income from her husband's pension, a little from her own, and the state pension. She feels she manages OK. She rates this area as 4.

Spirituality and Morality. She does not go to church although she was married in church. She rates this area as 3.

Compassion and Empathy. She has not really thought much about this area. She rates it as 4

Purpose. She sees herself as living out the rest of her life peacefully and with goodwill. If pushed she would rate this area as 2.

Chapter Seventeen: Balance: Reduce Distress or Develop Happiness?

There are times when our mood is low and distress presses, typically due to events that life has thrown at us. A relevant question is whether it is more appropriate to endeavour to increase happiness or to combat distress. Some examples are when we are:

- grieving,
- made redundant,
- being bullied or abused,
- imprisoned, or
- starting a painful and disabling illness.

Emotions generally do need to be expressed and worked through. Bottling up high pressures can lead to explosions. So, at times it can be more appropriate to have a good cry for example, and less relevant to try to find something to make us laugh. Distress can be viewed as a source or energy or prompt to take some action. It is a strong form of feedback. If you are fit enough, exercise can be a potent means of expressing the anger that often comes with distress. Peaceful activities like jogging, football, and golf, which include a kicking or hitting component can be helpful. Even rolling up a firm magazine and hitting a strong kitchen or outdoor bench can help. In some cases, it may well be appropriate to enter into some form of communication with the individual/s concerned, to move things along.

It can help a lot to express distress by talking. This is where companionship can be a great help. Associations for the recently bereaved or counselling may be appropriate for some people. If you are a friend of someone recently bereaved you can be a great help by letting them talk to you. Expect them to commonly repeat what they have told you before. Be empathic. They need to adjust to a new reality.

Time comes into the equation. So, if the low feeling persists and seems unlikely to be resolved soon, then it becomes appropriate to seek action to inject more happiness.

Chapter Eighteen: Internal Empowerment and Healing

In the course of progressing towards more happiness, there are a number of techniques that we can employ to help us on our way and to improve our mental and physical health, and our happiness. Battino (2000), in his excellent book '*Guided Imagery and Other Approaches to Healing*', page 18, writes:
   'If stress can suppress the immune system, why should not the opposite emotions such as joy, happiness, peace of mind, and relaxation strengthen the immune system.'
   He describes a number of researches confirming this viewpoint. In case you are in any doubt about the power of the mind just consider the following research by Luparello et al., as long ago as 1968:

A group of asthmatics were exposed to a nebulised saline solution (very fine droplets of salty water which are normally innocuous) and told that they were inhaling irritants or allergens.
47.5% of the group experienced substantially increased airway resistance.

Twelve subjects developed full-blown attacks.
They were relieved by the same saline solution when it was presented therapeutically.

So, the states of mind of these subjects were able to affect their health for the worse or the better. In the above case the individuals were responding to what they were told by those conducting the experiment.

Why not choose to use your own mind to deliberately help yourself?

You can create a helpful mental state, which is often dynamic (changing), in which as many of your senses as possible are engaged. That state is often referred to as an image. Importantly for our purpose, this is not just a visual image, although that frequently figures strongly in the state. I repeat: the image should involve as many of your senses as possible. Two helpful books that variously describe research or approaches in this area are:

Guided Imagery and Other Approaches to Healing by Rubin Battino, and
Creative Visualization: Using the Power of Your Imagination to Create What You Want in Your Life by Shakti Gawain.

For 'Imagery' and 'Visualization' in the context of those titles and this chapter, understand these generally to involve 'the use of as many senses as possible'.

Creating a Safe Place

A safe place, or 'safe haven' as Battino puts it, involves creating in one's mind a sensory image of a real or imaginary place in which one can feel at ease and safe. It is the basis of a number of approaches to relaxation, hypnosis, and therapy. It is likely to be very different for different people. It is helpful to explore a few ideas for yourself. It might involve a memory of an actual place you have been to, or the creation of one that seems particularly inviting. It is best that there will be no one else present, unless you choose to invite them in.

For some people, this might involve thoughts of a place by water. It might be in a quiet cove, by a calm blue sea, with a gentle warm sun, the scent of the sea, possibly the feel of an occasional light breeze, with the quiet lapping of small ripples at the edge of the sea, perhaps a bird sings in the green land behind, whilst you sip a refreshing drink.

For others, it might be in a lush Lake District valley, where a path broadens into a dell beside a gurgling stream not far from an ancient stone bridge. Wild flowers add a multitude of colours and fragrance. The weather will be comfortable, possibly a seagull calls as it soars above, whilst a pair of long-tailed tits land in a leafy bush. Further away you can see the valley narrowing as it climbs between grey screes and rock face. In the opposite direction, the valley widens to reveal woods and meadows as it approaches a lake.

Of course, it may well be that you will choose a dry destination. Some like to be on a hill or mountain top, giving a view of distant horizons in multiple hues, with a wonderful stillness in the air. Or, perhaps a quiet country meadow with nearby bushes and trees in full blossom would suit better.

Wherever appeals most to you, explore and soak up the effects of the view, scents in the air, pleasant gentle relaxing sensations on your body, peaceful yet delightful sounds, and even a calming taste in your mouth.

For the most benefit, practise approaching along a quiet path, with the wonder and calmness of your safe place developing as you get nearer to it. Spend a few minutes there. Then return at ease, refreshed, and better able to enjoy life and to be yourself.

Try using anchoring (described in the following subsection) to help you quickly access your safe place.

Anchoring
Anchoring is a technique developed in Neuro-Linguistic Programming, or NLP. It is a way to tie a helpful state of mind to

a trigger, commonly a body gesture, such as pressing thumb and little finger together on your left hand, or touching your right knee. When the gesture is repeated, the helpful state is quickly recalled. With practice this can be a powerful aid. Anchoring is an example of Pavlov's stimulus-response effect. It associates a sensory stimulus with the triggering of a feeling or behaviour. Typically, one uses a touch stimulus as the anchor. But have you ever seen someone licking an ice cream or sipping a cold drink and felt your mouth water? This is a similar effect with a visual trigger, cue, or anchor.

Try this with your safe place. Take a little time to use your mind to relax and meander along to your safe place. Let yourself be aware of the variety of sensory images: the colours and calming detail of the view, the delightful fragrances that you can smell, the interesting sounds that you can hear, the refreshing taste in your mouth, the pleasant sensations on and within your body, and the wonderful sense of comfort and ease. Intensify these sensations as much as you can, then bring your left thumb and little finger together with a firm gentle pressure for a few seconds. Then release. Repeat this three times. Later, try pressing your left thumb and little finger together and enjoy the sense of that pleasant relaxed state flooding through you.

You can use anchoring to induce a helpful feeling like confidence. The art is to recall a circumstance of the strongest feeling or behaviour you want, or to create an imaginary one. Enter as fully into the associated feelings as you can, letting yourself be aware of as many senses as possible. Intensify the feeling. Then apply the anchor. Then repeat twice. This can be a wonderful aid when you feel a need for a boost of confidence.

Relaxation
Deliberate planned relaxation can be very beneficial at times. There are number of things that you can do to optimise the experience, culminating in employing your safe place.

- Use a quiet location where you are unlikely to be disturbed.
- Get yourself into a comfortable position in an appropriate chair or bed.
- Overcome distracting thoughts by focussing on a simple object like a stone, or a flower.
- Count slowly backwards from ten to one.
- Focus on your gentle breathing. As you breath out, feel any anxiety, worry, or concern leaving you with each breath out. As you breath in, feel calm, peacefulness, and wellness entering and spreading through you.
- See and feel yourself approaching and entering your safe place.
- Relax and enjoy the sensations of your safe place.
- When you are ready, count upwards from one to ten, steadily becoming more alert and well with each increasing number. Return, feeling at ease and wonderfully refreshed.

Affirmations
Affirmations are positive statements that produce improved moods and help to develop subconscious attitudes. They help to produce outcomes that we desire, such as improved self-esteem and self-confidence. Affirmations are best kept short and address one desired outcome. They are framed in the positive

and the present. Avoid any negative. They are repeated several times. Examples are:

'I have stopped smoking and feel so much fitter.'

'I am enjoying eating smaller servings.'

'I am respected at work and talk confidently when I do a presentation.'

For best effects, it is helpful to recall occasions when you have had a good feeling about the topic and develop that mood to the best intensity you can whilst saying the affirmation. Affirmations are often included in self-hypnosis.

Self-hypnosis

Hypnosis is a wonderful way of using your subconscious mind to help yourself.

First you need to access your subconscious. It is found that this happens best when you are in a state of mind often called a trance. A trance, also known as an Altered State of Consciousness, can be defined as 'any mental state by an individual, or an observer, as being significantly different from "normal waking consciousness"' Edwards(2019).

It is actually very common. It is a state in which we are commonly very focussed and unaware of some external stimuli. For example, have you ever been intensely watching something on TV and been unaware of someone speaking to you until they shout or otherwise distract you? You would have been in an altered state then. At times, intense emotions or feelings can arise including excitement, or deep peace. It can also happen when one is very relaxed or meditating. When in such a state, it is possible for the conscious mind to be bypassed with words going directly to the subconscious mind. This is when affirmations can be made and suggestions given for behaviour after returning to normal consciousness.

Help Yourself to a Little More Happiness

To reach an appropriate altered state for self-hypnosis one commonly goes through a process of relaxation. This might be by developing the image of a safe place, or by progressively tightening and then relaxing a sequence of muscles in one's body, or by a breathing procedure. In the Appendices, there is a script that you can use for your own self-hypnosis. It is important to read it all through before trying it out. You will find that it works even better with more practice.

Chapter Nineteen: Conclusion

Thank you for letting me share an inner journey with you. The mind is a most wonderful entity and most of us use but a fraction of its potential.

I wish you well on your journey.

As comedian Dave Allen used to conclude:

'May your God go with you'.

Part Four: Appendices

Chapter Twenty: References and Further Reading

Ascher, D. (2019). What to do if you hate your boss. www.BBC/News, 6 October 2019, viewed 13 October 2019.

Battino, R. (2000). Guided Imagery and Other Approaches to Healing. Bancyfelin: Crown House Publishing.

Buzan, T. (2006). Use Your Head. Harlow: BBC Active.

Cameron, J. (2016). The Artist's Way. London: Macmillan.

Capacchione, L. (2002). The Creative Journal: Second Edition. Franklin Lakes: The Career Press.

Carr, A. (2011). Positive Psychology. 2nd ed. Hove: Routledge.

Csikszentmihalyi, M. (1997). Finding flow. The psychology of engagement in everyday life. New York: Basic Books.

Csikszentmihalyi, M. (2003). Good business, leadership, flow and the making of meaning. New York: Penguin Books.

de Waal, F.B.M. (2008). Putting the altruism back into altruism. The evolution of empathy. Annual Review of Psychology, 59. 279-300. In Carr, A. (2011).

Edwards, B.(1988). Drawing on the Artist Within. London: Fontana.

Edwards, B. (1993). Drawing on the Right Side of the Brain. London: HarperCollins.

Edwards, L. (2019) The other side of the valley. Alresford: O-Books.

Fordyce, M.W. (1983). A programme to increase happiness: Further studies. Journal of Counselling Psychology, 30(4). In Carr (2011).

Gawain, Shakti. (2002). Creative Visualization: Using the Power of Your Imagination to Create What You Want in Your Life. Novato: Nataraj Publishing.

Hartley, A. (2019). The importance of being moral. Posted 6 July 2016 , in www.psychologytoday.com, viewed 12 October 2019.

Luparello, T.J., Lyons, H.A., Bleeker E.R., & McFadden, E.R.. (1968). Influences of suggestion on airway reactivity in asthmatic subjects. Psychosomatic Medicine, 30:819-825. in Battino (2000).

Myers, D., Eid, M., & Larsen, R. J. (2008). Religion and human flourishing. In Eid, M. & Larsen, R. (Eds.) (2008). The science of subjective well-being. New York: Guilford Press.

Shernoff, D.J., & Csikszentmihalyi, M. (2009). Flow in schools: Cultivating engaged learners and optimal learning environments. In R. Gilman, E.S. Huebner, & M. J. Furlong (Eds.), Handbook of positive psychology in schools (pp131-145). New York: Routledge. In Carr, A. (2011).

Mind Mapping type Software

iThoughtsX, from www.toketa.com. Versions for iOS, Mac, and Windows.

Scapple, from www.literatureandlatte.com. Versions for Mac and Windows.

Chapter Twenty-One: Recreative Activities, Hobbies, and Sports

Amateur Dramatics
- Acting
- Front of House
- Props
- Scenery Construction

Amateur Radio
Angling
Art
- Acrylics
- Art Class
- Oils
- Painting
- Photography
- Pottery
- Sculpture
- Sketching
- Watercolour
- Wood Carving

Bee Keeping
Bell Ringing
Bird Watching
Bridge
Charity Work
Cheerleading
Chess

Collecting
- Fossils
- Minerals
- Sea Shells
- Stamps
- Stones

Dancing
- Ballet
- Ballroom
- Free
- Street
- Tap

Education. Find a Course/Offer to Teach
- Archaeology
- Art
- Business
- Electronics
- Engineering
- English
- Flower Arranging
- Foreign Language
- Geology
- History/Local History
- Music

- Science
- Vocational

Fashion Design
Flower Arranging
Flying
Gardening
Gliding
Jewellery Making
Jogging
Local Archaeology/History
Metal Detecting
Models and model making

- Aircraft
- Boats
- Buildings
- Cars
- Trains

Music

- Join a band/choir/orchestra
- Learn to play a musical instrument
- Sing

Orienteering
Pilates
Reading
Remote Control

- Aircraft
- Boats
- Cars

- Trains

Sport. Play, Coach, or Umpire/Referee
- Acrobatics
- Archery
- Athletics
- Badminton
- Basketball
- Billiards
- Bowls
- Canoeing
- Cricket
- Croquet
- Cycling
- Fencing
- Football
- Golf
- Gymnastics
- Hockey
- Horse Riding
- Judo
- Mixed Martial Arts
- Mountaineering
- Netball
- Rock Climbing

- Rowing
- Rugby
- Sailing
- Skiing and other snow sports
- Snooker
- Squash
- Swimming
- Table tennis
- Tennis

Vehicle Restoration
Voluntary work, e.g. in

- A Good Neighbour scheme
- A Hospital
- The Samaritans

Walking/Rambling
Woodworking
Writing

- Fiction
- Non-Fiction
- Plays
- Poetry

Yoga

Chapter Twenty-Two: Instructions for self-hypnosis

Read through these entire instructions before applying yourself to them.

USES
You can use self-hypnosis to help yourself in several ways: to improve your health or mood; to help lose weight or stop smoking; to explore what you want for the future; to take yourself into the future to experience achieving your goals; to ask for solutions to a problem; to ask for guidance or ideas about an important issue; or to lead in to relaxation or meditation.

PREPARING FOR SELF-HYPNOSIS
1. Decide what you want to use self-hypnosis for. It is best to concentrate on just one issue or application at a time.
2. Put this item into a *suggestion* which you will use. This should be a concise statement which is positive and in the present. For example: **I am relaxing and at ease / I feel confident / I am enjoying better breathing with cleaner lungs / Healing energy is reducing my pain / Healing love is making me better.**
3. Or you can prepare a *question*: **Please give me guidance in improving my relationship / What type of job will give me more fulfilment? / Please let me be aware what it will be like in six-month's-time when I have achieved ……**
4. Before going into Self-Hypnosis tell yourself the length of time for which you wish to remain relaxed, e.g. 5, 10, 15 minutes. If you wish to go to sleep immediately after the self-hypnosis tell yourself that you will go to sleep afterwards and that you will awake when it is appropriate.

TO ENTER SELF-HYPNOSIS
Tell yourself that you are now going to do SELF-HYPNOSIS.

1. Make yourself comfortable.

2. Close your eyes.

3. Take a deep breath in, being aware of a wonderful healing relaxing feeling entering you, of whatever colour and sound is most beautiful to you, and breathe out gently and slowly, allowing all stresses to leave you as you breathe out. Now just breathe gently and calmly allowing yourself to ease down comfortably and safely into a tranquil peaceful deep relaxation.

4. Slowly, in your mind, count down from 10 to 1, becoming aware how your muscles progressively relax throughout your body and sensing an occasional tingling of your skin as it eases gently, with each lower number drifting you steadily to calmness and peacefulness. When you reach number 1, allow yourself in your mind, to step into your own SAFE, BEAUTIFUL, HEALING PLACE of Deep Relaxation, Love, and Tranquillity, a place that is safe and secure, where no one else can enter without your permission. A place of beautiful scenery, wonderful sounds, treasured feelings, fragrant scents, and refreshing tastes. This is your own very special place where you can enjoy taking time out to simply be at peace, to allow joy, healing, confidence, love, strength, and goodwill, to flow into you. A place where, if you wish, you can explore what you would like for yourself, be aware of the steps, and contemplate yourself achieving your goals.

5. Here, you can simply give yourself your **positive suggestion**, or **ask your question**, or just **be at ease** and allow **healing and love to be with you**. Just focus on one issue in any one self-hypnosis.

TO END SELF-HYPNOSIS
(If you wish to go sleep after the self-hypnosis omit this section. Rather, tell yourself that it will turn into natural sleep from which you will awaken at the appropriate time.)

Slowly, in your mind, count up from 1 to 10, allowing your alertness, heart, and breathing to steadily pick up. When you get to 9: take a nice deep breath and smile. When you get to 10: open your eyes and feel refreshed and well.

PRACTICE
Self-hypnosis becomes more effective with practice. Use it to help with self-esteem, confidence, better sleep, and improved creativity, amongst many other opportunities for personal progress.

Printed in Poland
by Amazon Fulfillment
Poland Sp. z o.o., Wrocław